MICHAEL EBADAT

The Language of Fruits & Vegetables

Discover the Hidden Power of Nutrients for a Healthier Life

Contents

Introduction

The Forgotten Power of Nature's Gifts

In today's hectic world, many of us reach for what's quick and convenient regarding food. Processed snacks, fast food, and sugary treats fit better into our busy lives than a fresh salad or fruit. But what if I told you that the key to feeling better, having more energy, and even living longer could be as simple as adding more fruits and vegetables to your plate?

It's easy to forget just how powerful these natural foods are. For centuries, fruits and vegetables were the backbone of human diets. They provided the essential nutrients needed for survival, growth, and health. But as our diets have changed over time—replacing whole foods with processed options—we've also seen a rise in health problems like obesity, heart disease, and diabetes. And the sad truth is, that many of us aren't eating nearly enough fruits and vegetables to get the benefits they offer.

The good news is that nature still provides everything we need to nourish our bodies, and fruits and vegetables are among the most powerful allies in the fight for better health. These simple, whole foods are packed with vitamins, minerals, antioxidants, and fiber—things our bodies crave to function at their best. Adding more of them to your daily routine can help reduce the risk of chronic diseases, boost your immune system, increase your energy levels, and even improve your mood.

This book aims to help you rediscover the hidden potential of fruits and vegetables—not just as a way to fill your plate, but as a way to transform your health. We're going to dig into the science behind why these foods are so important, but more importantly, we're going to explore how easy and rewarding it can be to make them a bigger part of your life.

You don't need to become a nutrition expert or give up all your favorite foods to see results. Small changes, like swapping out a snack for a piece of fruit or adding more veggies to your dinner. Along the way, we'll address common concerns—whether it's worrying about cost, taste, or not knowing how to prepare certain foods—and give you simple, practical tips that fit into your busy life.

By the end of this journey, you'll see that fruits and vegetables aren't just a side dish—they can be a cornerstone of your overall well-being. Whether you're looking to improve your energy, manage your weight, prevent disease, or just feel better day to day, embracing these foods will help you get there.

We'll cover important questions, such as:

- Why are fruits and vegetables such a critical part of our health?
- What are the specific nutrients they offer, and how do they benefit our bodies?
- How can adding more fruits and veggies help prevent or even manage common diseases like diabetes, heart disease, and cancer?

The answers might surprise you. And they might just inspire you to see fruits and vegetables in a whole new light. Eating well doesn't have to be complicated or expensive, and it certainly doesn't have to be boring. In fact, by embracing the variety and vibrancy of plant-based foods, you're opening the door to a healthier, more fulfilling life.

So, let's get started. Together, we'll explore the hidden power of fruits and vegetables and discover how these natural gifts can lead to a happier, healthier you. It's time to reconnect with what nature has always provided us and take the first steps toward living better—one bite at a time.

1

Chapter 1

Fruits & Vegetables as Nutrient Powerhouses

When you think about eating healthier, what's the first thing that comes to mind? Probably something along the lines of "more fruits and vegetables." But why? Why do nutritionists, doctors, and health experts seem to be constantly pushing us to add more of these colorful, vibrant foods to our plates?

It turns out, there's a really good reason for that. Fruits and vegetables are like nature's multivitamins—packed with everything our bodies need to thrive. Whether it's boosting your energy, strengthening your immune system, or improving your heart health, these simple, whole foods are absolute powerhouses when it comes to nutrients. They're low in calories but high in the things that matter: vitamins, minerals, antioxidants, and fiber. The best part? They're delicious, versatile, and available in endless varieties, meaning there's something for everyone.

In this chapter, we'll explore what makes fruits and vegetables so special.

You'll learn about the different nutrients they contain and why they're so important for your health. By the end, you'll see why making room for more of these foods in your daily meals is one of the best decisions you can make for your body.

Why Fruits and Vegetables Matter

Think of fruits and vegetables as the MVPs of your diet. They may not always take center stage, but without them, your body simply can't perform at its best. While it's easy to reach for processed foods that are quick and convenient, those options often leave you feeling sluggish, and tired, and, over time, they can contribute to long-term health problems. On the other hand, fruits and vegetables give your body the fuel it craves to feel energized and stay healthy.

Not only do they provide essential vitamins and minerals, but they're also rich in fiber, which keeps your digestive system running smoothly and helps control your blood sugar. Plus, they're loaded with antioxidants—little molecules that fight off harmful substances in your body that can lead to inflammation, disease, and premature aging.

If you want to feel your best—both mentally and physically—it's hard to beat the impact of adding more fruits and vegetables to your diet.

What Are Macronutrients and Micronutrients?

Before we dive into the specifics, let's talk a little bit about the basics of nutrition. Your body needs two main types of nutrients: macronutrients and micronutrients.

Macronutrients—carbohydrates, proteins, and fats—are the big players. These provide energy and are found in all sorts of foods, from meat and dairy to grains and nuts.

Micronutrients, on the other hand, are the smaller, but equally important players. These are the vitamins and minerals that fruits and vegetables are packed with, and they play a huge role in keeping your body's systems running smoothly. While macronutrients fuel you, micronutrients make sure everything works the way it should.

Fruits and vegetables are a little bit of both. They're an excellent source of healthy carbohydrates and fiber (more on that in a bit), but their real magic comes from the vitamins, minerals, and antioxidants they offer. Let's look at some of the key nutrients you get when you load up on these powerhouse foods.

The Key Nutrients in Fruits and Vegetables

1. Fiber: The Quiet Hero

Fiber doesn't always get the attention it deserves, but it's essential for good health. Found in nearly all fruits and vegetables, fiber helps keep your digestive system happy and prevents problems like constipation. But that's not all—fiber can also help regulate blood sugar levels, making it a crucial ally for anyone dealing with diabetes or trying to prevent it.

Even better, fiber helps you feel full for longer, which can be a big help if you're trying to manage your weight. Instead of reaching for a sugary snack that will leave you hungry again in an hour, try an apple or a handful of carrots. You'll stay satisfied longer, and your body will thank you for the fiber boost.

Fiber-rich fruits and veggies include:

- Apples
- Broccoli
- Carrots
- Spinach
- Pears

2. Vitamin C: The Immune System's Best Friend

When the cold season rolls around, Vitamin C is the first thing many reach for—and with good reason! This essential vitamin, found in many fruits and vegetables, is a major player in supporting your immune system. It helps your body fight off infections and illness, so you can stay healthy and recover faster when you do get sick.

But Vitamin C does more than just protect you from colds. It also plays a key role in keeping your skin healthy, promoting wound healing, and even helping your body absorb iron from plant-based foods. So, next time you bite into an orange or a strawberry, know that you're doing more than just satisfying your sweet tooth—you're giving your body a serious health boost.

Vitamin C-rich foods include:

- Oranges
- Bell peppers
- Strawberries

- Kiwi
- Broccoli

3. Potassium: The Heart Protector

Potassium is another superstar mineral that fruits and vegetables deliver in spades. It's crucial for maintaining healthy blood pressure, supporting proper muscle function, and keeping your heart strong. If you're not getting enough potassium, you could be at risk for high blood pressure, muscle cramps, or even heart problems down the line.

The good news is that potassium is abundant in many fruits and vegetables, so it's easy to get your daily dose. By adding potassium-rich foods like bananas or sweet potatoes to your meals, you're giving your heart the protection it needs to keep you going strong.

Foods rich in potassium include:

- Bananas
- Sweet potatoes
- Spinach
- Avocados
- Tomatoes

4. Folate: For Cell Growth and Health

Folate, also known as Vitamin B9, is especially important for pregnant women because it helps support healthy cell growth and prevents birth defects. But it's not just for expectant mothers—folate is crucial for everyone, as it helps produce new cells and supports overall growth and development. If you're feeling tired or run down, it could be a sign that you're not getting enough folate in your diet.

Luckily, folate is found in abundance in leafy greens and other vegetables. By eating a salad packed with spinach, asparagus, and lentils, you're giving your body the nutrients it needs to stay strong and energized.

Folate-rich foods include:

- Leafy greens like spinach and kale
- Asparagus
- Citrus fruits
- Lentils
- Brussels sprouts

Variety Is Key: Eat the Rainbow

One of the best things about fruits and vegetables is their incredible variety. From the deep reds of tomatoes and strawberries to the bright oranges of carrots and sweet potatoes, the different colors of produce offer more than just visual appeal—they also signify different nutrients and health benefits.

That's why experts often recommend "eating the rainbow." By filling your plate with a colorful variety of fruits and vegetables, you'll ensure that you're getting a wide range of nutrients. For example:

- Red fruits and veggies like tomatoes and red peppers are high in lycopene, an antioxidant that supports heart health.
- Orange and yellow foods like carrots and mangoes are rich in beta-carotene, which is good for your eyes and skin.
- Green vegetables like spinach and broccoli are loaded with vitamins and minerals that support everything from bone health to immunity.
- Purple and blue foods like blueberries and eggplant are packed with anthocyanins, which help fight inflammation and protect your brain.
- By making a conscious effort to eat a variety of fruits and vegetables every day, you'll be giving your body all the nutrients it needs to stay healthy and strong.

Conclusion: Fruits and Vegetables as Your Daily Health Boost

It's clear that fruits and vegetables are more than just a side dish—they're a cornerstone of a healthy lifestyle. Packed with fiber, vitamins, minerals, and antioxidants, these foods support everything from heart health and digestion to immunity and energy. And the best part? They're delicious and easy to incorporate into your meals.

So, whether it's adding a handful of spinach to your smoothie, snacking on carrot sticks, or enjoying a fruit salad, there are endless ways to bring more fruits and vegetables into your diet. And as you do, you'll start to feel the difference—more energy, better digestion, and a stronger immune system.

In the next chapter, we'll dive even deeper into the specific vitamins and minerals found in fruits and vegetables, exploring how they work in your body and the best foods to get them from. But for now, remember: each bite of produce is a step toward a healthier, more vibrant life.

2

Chapter 2

Vitamins and Minerals – The Building Blocks of Health

You've probably heard it all your life: "Eat your fruits and vegetables—they're good for you!" But have you ever stopped to wonder why? What is it about these foods that make them so essential for your health? The answer lies in the vitamins and minerals they contain. These tiny nutrients may be small, but they are absolute powerhouses that help your body function properly every single day.

In this chapter, we're going to take a closer look at the specific vitamins and minerals found in fruits and vegetables and how they work to keep you feeling your best. By the end, you'll understand not just why they're important, but also how easy it is to get them into your daily meals—and why it's worth the effort.

Why Vitamins and Minerals Matter

Think of your body as a high-performance machine. Just like a car needs

12

fuel to run, your body needs nutrients to function at its best. And just as a car requires different types of fluids to keep its engine running smoothly—like oil, coolant, and gas—your body requires different vitamins and minerals to keep things humming along.

While macronutrients like carbs, fats, and proteins provide the energy your body uses, micronutrients— vitamins and minerals—are like the team that keeps everything running. They help your cells grow, fight off infections, and keep your organs, bones, and muscles in tip-top shape. If you don't get enough of these nutrients, your body can start to sputter—leading to problems like fatigue, weakened immunity, or even more serious health issues down the road.

The great news is that fruits and vegetables are some of the best sources of these vital nutrients. And because they come in natural, whole-food forms, your body can absorb and use them much more efficiently than from supplements.

Let's Talk Vitamins: What They Do and Where to Get Them:

1. Vitamin C: The Immune System's Superhero

You've probably heard of Vitamin C—it's the go-to vitamin when you feel a cold coming on. But Vitamin C does so much more than just fight off colds. It's a powerful antioxidant, meaning it helps protect your cells from damage. It's also key for making collagen, which keeps your skin, bones, and tissues strong. Plus, it supports your immune system, helping you bounce back from illness more quickly.

Getting enough Vitamin C from your diet can be as simple as enjoying a juicy orange or snacking on bell peppers. And yes, even those strawberries you love are packed with this vitamin!

Where to find Vitamin C:

- Oranges
- Strawberries
- Bell peppers
- Kiwi
- Broccoli

2. Vitamin A: Your Eyes' Best Friend

Vitamin A is a real multitasker. It's famous for being essential for your vision, especially for seeing in low light. But that's not all—Vitamin A also helps keep your skin and immune system healthy. The body gets Vitamin A from beta-carotene, a compound found in many orange and yellow fruits and vegetables. So when you're eating sweet potatoes or carrots, you're doing your eyes and your whole body a favor.

Where to find Vitamin A (beta-carotene):

- Carrots
- Sweet potatoes
- Mangoes
- Pumpkin
- Spinach

3. Folate (Vitamin B9): The Cell Builder

Folate (also called Vitamin B9) is crucial for cell growth and repair. It's especially important for pregnant women because it helps prevent birth defects. But folate is important for everyone—it supports red blood cell production, which helps keep you energized and feeling your best. A lack of folate can lead to fatigue, anemia, and a weakened immune system. Luckily, leafy greens and avocados are excellent sources.

Where to find folate:

- Leafy greens (spinach, kale)
- Asparagus
- Avocados
- Brussels sprouts
- Oranges

4. Vitamin K: The Bone and Blood Buddy

Vitamin K may not be as well-known as some other vitamins, but it plays a critical role in your body. It helps your blood clot properly, so if you ever cut yourself, you'll stop bleeding. It's also key for bone health, helping your body use calcium to build strong bones and prevent osteoporosis. Dark leafy greens like kale and spinach are packed with Vitamin K, making them great choices for your blood and bones.

Where to find Vitamin K:

- Kale
- Spinach
- Swiss chard
- Broccoli
- Green beans

Essential Minerals You Get from Fruits and Vegetables

Just like vitamins, minerals are a must for your body's health. They help keep everything from your heart to your muscles to your bones in good working order. Let's look at some of the most important ones found in fruits and vegetables.

1. Potassium: The Heart Health Guardian

Potassium is a rockstar when it comes to keeping your heart healthy. It helps regulate your blood pressure by balancing the effects of sodium. If you're not getting enough potassium, you could be putting yourself at risk for high blood pressure and heart disease. Potassium also helps your muscles work properly and prevents cramps. And the good news? Many fruits and vegetables, like bananas and avocados, are packed with this essential mineral.

Where to find potassium:

- Bananas
- Sweet potatoes
- Avocados
- Tomatoes

• Spinach

2. Magnesium: The Muscle and Nerve Helper

Magnesium is one of those minerals that's involved in just about everything your body does. It helps regulate your muscles and nerves, keeps your heart steady, and supports bone health. Magnesium is also important for converting the food you eat into energy. Without enough magnesium, you might experience muscle cramps, fatigue, or even more serious health issues. Leafy greens and nuts are excellent sources of this vital mineral.

Where to find magnesium:

• Spinach
• Swiss chard
• Almonds
• Avocados
• Black beans

3. Calcium: The Bone Builder

When you think of calcium, you probably think of milk. But did you know that many vegetables, particularly dark leafy greens, are also great sources of calcium? Calcium is essential for building and maintaining strong bones and teeth, and it also helps your muscles and nerves function properly. Getting enough calcium is especially important as you age, helping to prevent osteoporosis.

Where to find calcium:

- Broccoli
- Kale
- Collard greens
- Figs
- Oranges

Why Whole Foods Are Better Than Supplements

It might be tempting to reach for a multivitamin to get your daily dose of vitamins and minerals, but studies show that getting your nutrients from whole foods like fruits and vegetables is much more effective. Why? Whole foods don't just provide individual nutrients—they offer a whole package of vitamins, minerals, fiber, and antioxidants that work together to give your body what it needs.

For example, when you eat an orange, you're not just getting Vitamin C—you're also getting fiber, water, and other nutrients that help your body absorb and use that Vitamin C more effectively. It's like a team effort: all the parts of the food work together to support your health.

Conclusion: Make Vitamins and Minerals Part of Your Daily Routine

Vitamins and minerals may seem small, but they have a huge impact on your health. From keeping your immune system strong to ensuring your muscles, bones, and heart function properly, these nutrients are the building blocks that help your body thrive. And the best way to get them? By eating a variety of fruits and vegetables every day.

Remember, it's not about perfection—it's about progress. Whether you start by adding a few more veggies to your dinner plate or swapping a sugary snack for a piece of fruit, every little step brings you closer to a healthier, more vibrant you.

In the next chapter, we'll explore the world of antioxidants and phytochemicals—those powerful compounds in fruits and vegetables that protect your body from disease and keep you feeling your best.

3

Chapter 3

Phytochemicals – The Hidden Warriors

You've probably heard plenty about vitamins and minerals, but there's a group of nutrients in fruits and vegetables that often gets overlooked: phytochemicals. Think of these compounds as the secret superheroes of the plant world. They're not considered essential like vitamins (meaning you won't get sick if you don't have them), but their ability to protect your health is nothing short of amazing.

Phytochemicals are the hidden warriors in fruits and vegetables, working behind the scenes to help your body fend off damage, inflammation, and disease. They're like little bodyguards that come to the rescue when things go wrong, protecting you from illnesses like heart disease, diabetes, and even cancer.

In this chapter, we're going to take a closer look at what phytochemicals are, why they're so important, and how you can easily get more of them into your diet. By the end, you'll see just how powerful these plant compounds are—and why adding more fruits and veggies to your plate is one of the best things you can do for your health.

What Exactly Are Phytochemicals?

At first glance, "phytochemicals" might sound complicated, but they're just natural compounds found in plants. The word "phyto" means plant, and these chemicals are part of a plant's defense system. They protect plants from environmental threats like pests, disease, and UV radiation. But when we eat these plants, these same phytochemicals start protecting us.

While you won't get a deficiency from not having enough phytochemicals (like you would with a lack of Vitamin C or calcium), they offer huge benefits when it comes to long-term health. They're packed with antioxidants and anti-inflammatory properties that help protect your body from the inside out. From keeping your cells safe from damage to supporting your immune system, phytochemicals do some pretty incredible work behind the scenes.

The best part? They're everywhere. Fruits, vegetables, nuts, and seeds are all rich in phytochemicals, and each type of food offers a different mix of these compounds. This is why it's so important to eat a variety of plant-based foods—the more variety, the more health benefits you'll get.

The Power of Phytochemicals: Different Types and Their Benefits

There are thousands of different phytochemicals, but don't worry—you don't need to memorize them all. What's important is knowing what they do and where to find them. Let's break down a few of the most important types of phytochemicals and how they can help you stay healthy.

1. Flavonoids: The Ultimate Antioxidants

Flavonoids are like the superheroes of the antioxidant world. Antioxidants help protect your cells from damage caused by free radicals—unstable molecules that can lead to inflammation, aging, and disease. By fighting off these harmful molecules, flavonoids play a key role in reducing your risk of chronic diseases like cancer and heart disease.

Different flavonoids offer different benefits. For example, some help reduces inflammation, while others improve heart health by lowering blood pressure and cholesterol. So, the next time you're snacking on some berries or sipping green tea, know that you're giving your body a serious health boost.

Where to find flavonoids:

- Berries (blueberries, strawberries)
- Citrus fruits (oranges, lemons)
- Apples
- Onions
- Green tea

2. Carotenoids: Eye Health and Cancer Fighters

Carotenoids are what give fruits and vegetables their vibrant red, orange, and yellow colors. They're also amazing at protecting your cells from damage. One of the most famous carotenoids is beta-carotene, which your body converts into Vitamin A—essential for good vision, especially in low light.

Carotenoids aren't just good for your eyes, though. Studies have shown that they can also reduce the risk of certain cancers and boost your immune system. So when you're munching on carrots or tomatoes, you're doing much more than enjoying a tasty snack—you're helping your body fight disease.

Where to find carotenoids:

- Carrots
- Sweet potatoes
- Tomatoes
- Spinach
- Bell peppers

3. Polyphenols: Protecting Your Heart and Brain

Polyphenols are another group of phytochemicals with powerful antioxidant properties. They're especially good at protecting your heart, helping to lower blood pressure and reduce inflammation in your blood vessels. Polyphenols also help protect your brain and may reduce the risk of neurodegenerative diseases like Alzheimer's.

One of the most famous polyphenols is resveratrol, found in red grapes and, yes, wine. It's part of the reason why moderate wine consumption is often linked to heart health benefits. But don't worry—you don't need to drink wine to get your polyphenol fix. Plenty of other foods, like berries and nuts, are also rich in these heart-healthy compounds.

Where to find polyphenols:

- Red grapes
- Blueberries
- Apples
- Walnuts
- Dark chocolate

4. Glucosinolates: Natural Cancer Fighters

Glucosinolates are found primarily in cruciferous vegetables like broccoli, cabbage, and kale. They're known for their ability to help detoxify your body and encourage the death of cancer cells. Studies suggest that eating more glucosinolates may reduce your risk of cancers like colon, lung, and breast cancer.

And while glucosinolates are responsible for the slightly bitter taste of these veggies, they're worth it for the incredible health benefits they offer. So, if you've been avoiding Brussels sprouts, it might be time to give them another shot.

Where to find glucosinolates:

- Broccoli
- Kale

- Cabbage
- Brussels sprouts
- Radishes

5. Anthocyanins: Keeping Your Heart and Skin Healthy

Anthocyanins give red, purple, and blue fruits and vegetables their bold colors. These phytochemicals are known for their antioxidant properties, and they've been linked to improved heart health. They help reduce inflammation and oxidative stress, both of which are important for preventing heart disease.

But anthocyanins aren't just good for your heart—they're also great for your skin. They help protect against damage caused by UV radiation, which can lead to premature aging and wrinkles. So, the next time you're enjoying some blueberries or purple cabbage, know that you're giving both your heart and your skin some love.

Where to find anthocyanins:

- Blueberries
- Blackberries
- Red cabbage
- Purple sweet potatoes
- Cherries

Phytochemicals and Disease Prevention: How They Help Keep You Healthy

Phytochemicals are more than just antioxidants—they're powerful protectors that can help prevent some of the most common chronic diseases.

1. Lowering Cancer Risk

Many phytochemicals, like glucosinolates and carotenoids, have been shown to reduce the risk of certain types of cancer. They do this by protecting your cells from damage, encouraging the death of cancer cells, and even helping your body detoxify carcinogens (cancer-causing substances). So, when you load up on broccoli, carrots, and other colorful veggies, you're giving your body a fighting chance against cancer.

2. Supporting Heart Health

Flavonoids, polyphenols, and anthocyanins are all great for your heart. They help reduce inflammation, lower cholesterol levels, and keep your blood pressure in check. Studies have shown that people who eat more fruits and vegetables—especially those rich in these phytochemicals— have a lower risk of heart disease and stroke.

3. Protecting Your Brain

Phytochemicals, particularly polyphenols, have been shown to protect the brain from oxidative stress and inflammation, both of which can contribute to cognitive decline as we age. Some studies even suggest that eating a diet rich in phytochemicals can help improve memory and reduce the risk of neurodegenerative diseases like Alzheimer's.

How to Get More Phytochemicals in Your Diet

The good news is that getting more phytochemicals in your diet doesn't have to be hard. It can be as simple as eating a variety of fruits and vegetables every day. Here are a few easy ways to boost your phytochemical intake:

- Eat the rainbow: Aim to fill your plate with fruits and vegetables from all the color groups. The more colors you eat, the more phytochemicals you're getting.
- Snack smart: Keep berries and nuts on hand for easy, nutrient-packed snacks.
- Try new veggies: Add more cruciferous vegetables like kale, broccoli, and Brussels sprouts to your meals. These veggies are packed with cancer-fighting glucosinolates.
- Enjoy dark chocolate: Yes, you read that right! Dark chocolate is a great source of polyphenols, so you can indulge your sweet tooth and boost your health at the same time. Just remember to choose varieties with a high cocoa content.

Conclusion: Phytochemicals – The Unsung Heroes of Your Diet

Phytochemicals may not be as well-known as vitamins and minerals, but their benefits are just as powerful. These hidden warriors protect your cells, reduce inflammation, and help prevent diseases like cancer, heart disease, and even cognitive decline. And the best part? You don't need to overhaul your diet to reap the benefits. By simply eating a variety of fruits, vegetables, nuts, and seeds every day, you can easily give your body the phytochemicals it needs to stay healthy and strong.

In the next chapter, we'll dive into how fruits and vegetables help prevent specific diseases like heart disease, cancer, and diabetes, and how small changes to your diet can make a big difference.

4

Chapter 4

Fruits & Vegetables for Disease Prevention

We've all heard the saying, "An apple a day keeps the doctor away," and while that might sound like an old cliché, it holds more truth than you might think. Fruits and vegetables aren't just colorful, delicious additions to our meals—they are some of the most powerful tools we have to keep ourselves healthy and fight off diseases. From heart disease and cancer to diabetes and obesity, a diet rich in fruits and vegetables can make a huge difference in keeping your body in tip-top shape.

In this chapter, we're going to dive into how these plant-based superfoods help protect your body from common, chronic diseases. We'll talk about how the nutrients, fiber, and natural compounds in fruits and vegetables work together to shield your health. By the end of this chapter, you'll see that these foods aren't just side dishes—they're true life savers.

How What We Eat Affects Our Health

Think about your body like a car. If you fuel it with the right stuff, it runs smoothly and gets you where you need to go. But if you fill it with junk, it sputters, slows down, and eventually, parts start to break down. The same thing happens with our bodies. What we eat plays a huge role in how well our bodies perform and how long we can keep cruising through life without hitting health speed bumps.

Diets that are full of processed foods, sugary snacks, and unhealthy fats have been linked to an increased risk of developing serious health problems like heart disease, diabetes, and cancer. On the other hand, a diet that's rich in fruits and vegetables helps your body fight off these diseases by providing essential nutrients and protecting your cells from damage.

It's like giving your body the best fuel possible, ensuring it runs efficiently for years to come. And the good news? You don't need to make drastic changes. Simply eating more fruits and vegetables can go a long way in helping your body stay healthy.

Fruits and Vegetables: Your Heart's Best Friend

Heart disease is the leading cause of death around the world, but here's the good news—it's also one of the most preventable. One of the easiest ways to protect your heart is by adding more fruits and vegetables to your meals. Here's why:

1. Lowering Your Blood Pressure

High blood pressure, or hypertension, is one of the biggest risk factors for heart disease and stroke. Thankfully, fruits and vegetables are packed with potassium, a mineral that helps your body balance the effects of sodium (which can raise blood pressure). When you eat potassium-rich foods like bananas, spinach, and sweet potatoes, you're giving your blood vessels the signal to relax and lower your blood pressure—keeping your heart from working too hard.

2. Reducing Bad Cholesterol

Many fruits and veggies are rich in soluble fiber, which helps lower "bad" LDL cholesterol. High cholesterol can cause plaque to build up in your arteries, which can lead to heart attacks. Fiber acts like a sponge, soaking up cholesterol in your digestive system and helping to get rid of it before it causes harm. Apples, carrots, and beans are excellent sources of this heart-protecting fiber.

3. Fighting Inflammation

Chronic inflammation is a major contributor to heart disease. Thankfully, many fruits and vegetables contain anti-inflammatory compounds that help protect your blood vessels. Berries, in particular, are loaded with flavonoids, which reduce inflammation and keep your heart in good shape. So, next time you snack on blueberries or strawberries, know that you're doing something great for your heart.

Fruits and Vegetables: Your Body's Cancer Fighters

Cancer is one of those diseases that can feel especially scary, but there are ways to reduce your risk—and eating more fruits and vegetables is one of the most powerful. How exactly do these foods help protect us from cancer?

1. Neutralizing Free Radicals

Free radicals are unstable molecules that can damage cells and lead to cancer. Fortunately, fruits and vegetables are packed with antioxidants, which help neutralize these harmful molecules before they can cause problems. For example, carotenoids, found in carrots and sweet potatoes, and flavonoids, found in berries and leafy greens, are especially effective at protecting your cells from damage.

2. Detoxifying Your Body

Cruciferous vegetables—like broccoli, kale, and Brussels sprouts—contain special compounds called glucosinolates, which help your body detoxify carcinogens (substances that can cause cancer). These veggies help your body break down and eliminate harmful chemicals before they can do any damage, making them a powerful ally in cancer prevention.

3. Supporting Healthy Cell Growth

Some fruits and vegetables are rich in folate, a B vitamin is crucial for proper cell growth and division. Folate, found in leafy greens, citrus fruits, and avocados, helps your body make and repair DNA, which is key for preventing cells from turning cancerous. It's like giving your body the tools it needs to keep your cells healthy and functioning properly.

Preventing and Managing Diabetes with Fruits and Vegetables

Diabetes is a growing problem worldwide, especially Type 2 diabetes, which is often related to diet and lifestyle. Luckily, eating more fruits and vegetables can play a huge role in both preventing and managing this condition.

1. Stabilizing Blood Sugar Levels

The fiber in fruits and vegetables helps slow down how quickly your body absorbs sugar, which prevents those big spikes and crashes in blood sugar that can lead to insulin resistance. Foods like apples, pears, and leafy greens are excellent for helping you maintain stable blood sugar levels throughout the day.

2. Reducing Insulin Resistance

Certain vegetables, like spinach, kale, and other leafy greens, are high in magnesium, which has been shown to improve insulin sensitivity. This means your body can use insulin more effectively, helping to prevent or manage Type 2 diabetes. Eating a diet rich in these veggies is like giving your body a natural way to keep blood sugar under control.

3. Managing Weight

Carrying extra weight is one of the main risk factors for diabetes, but fruits and vegetables can help with that too. They're low in calories but high in nutrients and fiber, which helps you feel full without overeating. By filling your plate with fruits and veggies, you can manage your weight and keep your blood sugar in check at the same time.

Keeping Obesity at Bay with Fruits and Vegetables

Obesity is linked to many chronic diseases, but one of the easiest—and tastiest—ways to keep it at bay is by eating more fruits and vegetables. Here's how they help:

1. Low in Calories, High in Nutrients

Fruits and vegetables are naturally low in calories but packed with nutrients. This means you can eat larger portions without consuming too many calories. So, whether you're snacking on cucumbers or filling up on a big salad, you can satisfy your hunger without overdoing it on calories.

2. Keeping You Full and Satisfied

The fiber in fruits and vegetables doesn't just help with digestion—it also helps you feel full and satisfied. This makes it easier to eat less overall, which can help you maintain a healthy weight. Plus, starting meals with a salad or veggie-packed soup can fill you up, so you're less likely to overeat the higher-calorie parts of your meal.

3. Encouraging Better Eating Habits

The more fruits and vegetables you add to your diet, the less room you'll have for processed, high-calorie foods. Over time, this leads to healthier eating habits that stick, helping you maintain a balanced diet and a healthy weight without feeling deprived.

Conclusion: Prevention Is the Best Medicine

At the end of the day, the old saying rings true—"an apple a day really can keep the doctor away." Fruits and vegetables are so much more than just a tasty part of your meal—they're some of the most powerful tools we have for preventing chronic diseases. Whether you're looking to protect your heart, reduce your cancer risk, manage your blood sugar, or keep your weight in check, these plant-based superfoods are your body's best defense.

And the best part? You don't need to make drastic changes. Simply adding more fruits and vegetables to your plate every day can make a huge difference. In the next chapter, we'll explore practical tips and tricks to help you easily incorporate more of these disease-fighting foods into your life.

5

Chapter 5

Practical Tips for Incorporating More Fruits & Vegetables

We all know that fruits and vegetables are good for us, but let's be real—sometimes it feels like a challenge to get enough of them into our meals. Whether it's because we're too busy, not sure how to prepare them, or think they're too expensive, making fruits and veggies a bigger part of our diet can seem like a struggle.

But here's the good news: it doesn't have to be hard. With just a few simple tweaks to your routine, you can easily up your intake of these nutrient-packed foods and make them a regular part of your life. In this chapter, we're going to talk about some super practical ways to sneak more fruits and vegetables into your day—whether you're cooking at home, grabbing a snack, or even eating out. By the end, you'll have some easy, realistic strategies to help you enjoy more of these delicious, health-boosting foods without feeling overwhelmed.

Start Small and Build from There

If the idea of overhauling your diet feels intimidating, don't worry—you don't need to change everything overnight. The best way to get started is to make small, manageable changes. Instead of trying to double your veggie intake all at once, aim to add just one extra serving of fruits or vegetables a day. Once you get used to that, add another, and so on. Slow and steady wins the race, and before you know it, you'll be eating way more fruits and veggies without even thinking about it.

Here are some super simple ways to get started:

Add veggies to breakfast: Throw a handful of spinach into your morning smoothie, or toss some chopped bell peppers or mushrooms into your scrambled eggs.

Snack on fruit: Keep an apple or banana within arm's reach for an easy, grab-and-go snack.

Switch outsides: When you're making lunch or dinner, swap out the chips or fries for a side salad, roasted veggies, or even a piece of fruit.

These little changes add up, and they're a great way to build healthier habits without feeling like you're making a huge effort.

Let Vegetables Take Center Stage

For a lot of us, vegetables are usually the sidekick on our plate, while meat or carbs are the main event. But what if you flipped the script? One of the easiest ways to eat more veggies is to make them the star of your meal. Think of it as giving veggies their moment to shine!

Here are some ideas to make vegetables the star of the show:

Veggie-based main dishes: Try making meals where vegetables are the main ingredient. Think stir-fries, grain bowls, or hearty salads. Mix in different kinds of vegetables to add variety and flavor.

Go meatless for a meal: Pick a day of the week to go plant-based. Try a veggie-loaded pasta, a vegetable curry, or a roasted veggie tray. These dishes are often just as filling and satisfying as their meat-based counterparts.

Sneak veggies into your favorites: Add extra vegetables to meals you already love. Toss spinach or zucchini into your pasta sauce, mix peppers, and onions into your tacos, or pile extra veggies on your pizza. The more you make veggies the focus of your meals, the easier it becomes to eat more of them—and it can be a lot of fun trying new combinations and flavors.

Keep It Simple: Quick and Easy Ways to Add More Veggies

One of the biggest hurdles people face when trying to eat more fruits and vegetables is the time it takes to prepare them. But here's a secret: it doesn't have to take long at all. Many fruits and veggies are ready to eat with minimal prep, and there are plenty of ways to make things even easier.

Here are some time-saving tips to get more fruits and veggies into your meals:

- **Eat them raw:** Many vegetables, like carrots, cucumbers, and bell peppers, are delicious raw. Just chop them up and enjoy them with a dip or add them to a salad—no cooking required.
- **Pre-cut for the week:** Spend a few minutes at the start of the week chopping up vegetables like celery, bell peppers, and carrots. Store them in containers so they're ready for snacking or tossing into a stir-fry or salad.
- **Buy pre-cut or frozen:** Don't have time to prep? No problem!

Pre-cut or frozen vegetables are just as nutritious and can be real time-savers. Keep a bag of frozen broccoli or mixed veggies on hand for quick meals.

- **Roast a big batch:** Roasting vegetables like sweet potatoes, Brussels sprouts, or cauliflower is an easy way to prepare a lot at once. Roast them in big batches, and use them throughout the week in salads, sandwiches, or as a side dish.

These tips make it easier to fit more veggies into your meals, even when life gets busy.

Snack Smarter with Fruits and Veggies

If you're someone who loves to snack (and who doesn't?), this is a perfect opportunity to sneak more fruits and veggies into your day. Instead of reaching for chips or cookies, switch things up with healthy, produce-packed snacks.

Here are some easy, tasty snack ideas:

- **Fruit with nut butter:** Slice up an apple or banana and pair it with peanut or almond butter for a snack that's both filling and delicious.
- **Veggies and hummus**: Cut up cucumbers, carrots, and bell peppers, and dip them in hummus or guacamole for a tasty, nutrient-packed snack.
- **Fruit salad:** Chop up a variety of fruits—whatever you have on hand—and keep them in the fridge for a quick, refreshing snack. You can sprinkle some nuts or seeds on top for extra crunch.
- **Smoothies:** Blend up a smoothie with your favorite fruits and

throw in a handful of spinach or kale for an added veggie boost. Smoothies are an easy way to get multiple servings of fruits and vegetables in one go.

Making smart snack choices is an easy and delicious way to increase your fruit and vegetable intake throughout the day.

Shop Smarter and Save Time and Money

One of the biggest myths about fruits and vegetables is that they're too expensive. While it's true that some produce can be pricey, there are plenty of ways to shop smarter and get more bang for your buck when buying fruits and veggies.

Here are a few tips to help you save time and money:

- Buy in season: Fruits and vegetables are usually cheaper when they're in season, and they often taste better, too. Check what's in season in your area and focus on those foods for the best deals.
- Go frozen: Frozen fruits and vegetables are often more affordable than fresh, and they're just as nutritious. Keep frozen berries, spinach, peas, and other veggies on hand for quick, easy meals.
- Buy in bulk: Vegetables like carrots, potatoes, and onions can last a long time if stored properly, so buying them in bulk can save you money in the long run.
- Shop local: Farmers markets and local produce stands can offer fresh, seasonal produce at lower prices than grocery stores. Plus, you're supporting local farmers!
- Store brands: Store-brand frozen or canned vegetables are often

cheaper than name brands, and they're just as good.

With a little bit of planning, you can easily stock up on fruits and veggies without breaking the bank.

Sneak in More Veggies When Eating Out

Eating out doesn't mean you have to give up on your healthy eating goals. There are plenty of ways to sneak more fruits and vegetables into your meals, even when you're ordering takeout or dining out at a restaurant.

Here's how to do it:

- **Pick veggie-heavy dishes:** Look for meals that feature vegetables, like salads, stir-fries, or grain bowls. These dishes are often loaded with flavor and packed with nutrients.
- **Add extra veggies:** Don't be shy about asking for extra vegetables with your meal. Whether it's adding spinach to your sandwich or an extra side of steamed veggies, most restaurants are happy to accommodate.
- **Swap sides:** When your meal comes with fries or chips, ask to swap them out for a side salad, steamed veggies, or fruit. It's an easy way to add more produce to your meal.
- **Go for fruit-based desserts:** If you're craving something sweet, opt for fresh fruit or a fruit-based dessert instead of heavier, sugary treats. Many restaurants offer fruit as a lighter dessert option.

Eating out doesn't have to derail your efforts to eat more fruits and veggies—you can make healthy choices anywhere.

Get the Whole Family Involved

Eating more fruits and vegetables can be fun for the whole family. Getting kids (or even adults!) involved in meal prep and experimenting with new fruits and veggies can help create healthy habits that stick. Plus, when everyone's involved, they're more likely to enjoy what they're eating.

Here are some fun ways to get the family excited about fruits and veggies:

- Pick a new veggie each week: Make it a game to try one new fruit or vegetable each week. Let the kids pick something new at the store, and then find a fun recipe to try together.
- Get creative: Arrange fruits and veggies into fun shapes, like smiley faces or animals, to make them more appealing—especially for picky eaters.
- Let the kids help: Kids are more likely to eat fruits and veggies if they help prepare them. Get them involved in washing, peeling, or chopping, and watch how excited they get to eat their creations.

Making fruits and vegetables fun can help your family develop lifelong healthy eating habits.

Conclusion: Small Steps to a Healthier You

Incorporating more fruits and vegetables into your diet doesn't have to be complicated. It's about making small, simple changes—like adding a side salad to dinner or grabbing a piece of fruit for a snack. These little tweaks add up over time and make a big difference in your health.

You don't need to be perfect or change everything at once. Just take it one step at a time, enjoy the process, and remember that every little bit counts. The goal is progress, not perfection. So, start small, keep it simple, and watch as these healthy habits become second nature.

6

Conclusion

Embracing a Healthier, Plant-Powered Life

By now, you've learned how incredible fruits and vegetables can be for your health. They boost your immune system, help prevent diseases, and even improve your energy and mood. The best part? Eating more of them doesn't have to be difficult or overwhelming. It's about making small, manageable changes that fit into your daily life—little by little, they'll add up to big results.

The beauty of this journey is that it's not about being perfect. You don't need to make massive changes overnight. Start by adding an extra serving of veggies to dinner, grabbing a piece of fruit for a snack, or experimenting with new recipes that make plants the star of the meal. These small steps make a huge difference over time, and soon enough, you'll notice how much better you feel.

Remember, this isn't a race—it's a lifestyle. There will be days when you eat more fruits and veggies, and others when you don't, and that's okay. What's important is that you're making progress. It's about enjoying the process, finding what works for you, and being kind to yourself along the way.

Not only will you be improving your physical health by eating more plant-based foods, but you're also doing something good for the environment. A plant-powered diet has a lighter environmental impact, making it a win-win for you and the planet.

So, as you move forward, take pride in every small step you make. Whether it's a vibrant salad for lunch or a fruit-packed smoothie for breakfast, know that you're taking control of your health one meal at a time. You've got all the tools to live a healthier, plant-powered life—now it's time to enjoy it!

7

Resources

Vegetables and fruits. (2024, May 9). The Nutrition Source. https://www.hsph.harvard.edu/nutritionsource/what-should-you-eat/vegetables-and-fruits/

World Health Organization: WHO. (2020, April 29). *Healthy diet.* https://www.who.int/news-room/fact-sheets/detail/healthy-diet

Office of Dietary Supplements - Nutrient Recommendations and Databases. (n.d.). https://ods.od.nih.gov/HealthInformation/nutrientrecommendations.aspx

Office of Dietary Supplements - Dietary supplements: What you need to know. (n.d.). https://ods.od.nih.gov/factsheets/WYNTK-Consumer/

Nutrition and Healthy Eating. (n.d.). SNAP Education Connection. https://snaped.fns.usda.gov/resources/nutrition-education-materials/nutrition-and-healthy-eating

American Heart Association. (23 C.E., October 26). *How to Eat More Fruit and Vegetables.* Retrieved September 29, 2024, from https://www.heart.org/en/healthy-living/healthy-eating/add-color/how-to-eat-more-fruits-and-vegetables

American Institute of Cancer Research. (20 C.E., January 26).

Wholegrains, vegetables & fruit. Retrieved September 29, 2024, from https://www.aicr.org/research/the-continuous-update-project/wholegrains-vegetables-fruit/

47